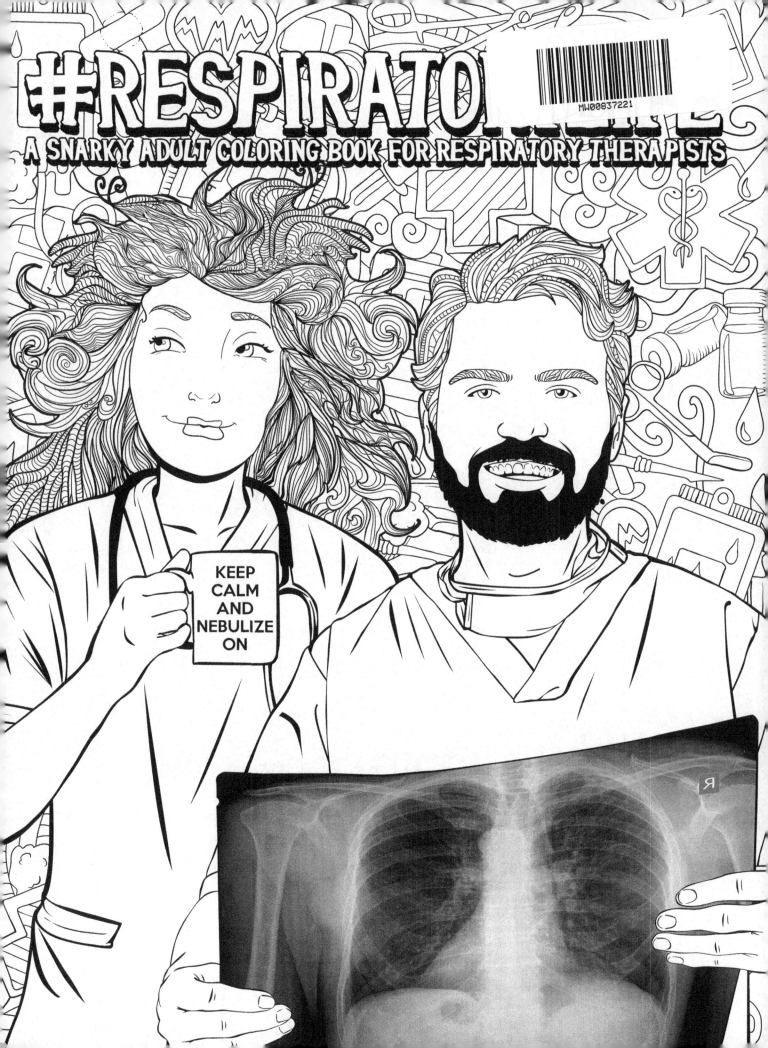

@papeteriebleu

Papeterie Bleu

Shop our other books at
www.pbleu.com

Wholesale distribution through Ingram Content Group
www.ingramcontent.com/publishers/distribution/wholesale

For questions and customer service, email us at
support@pbleu.com

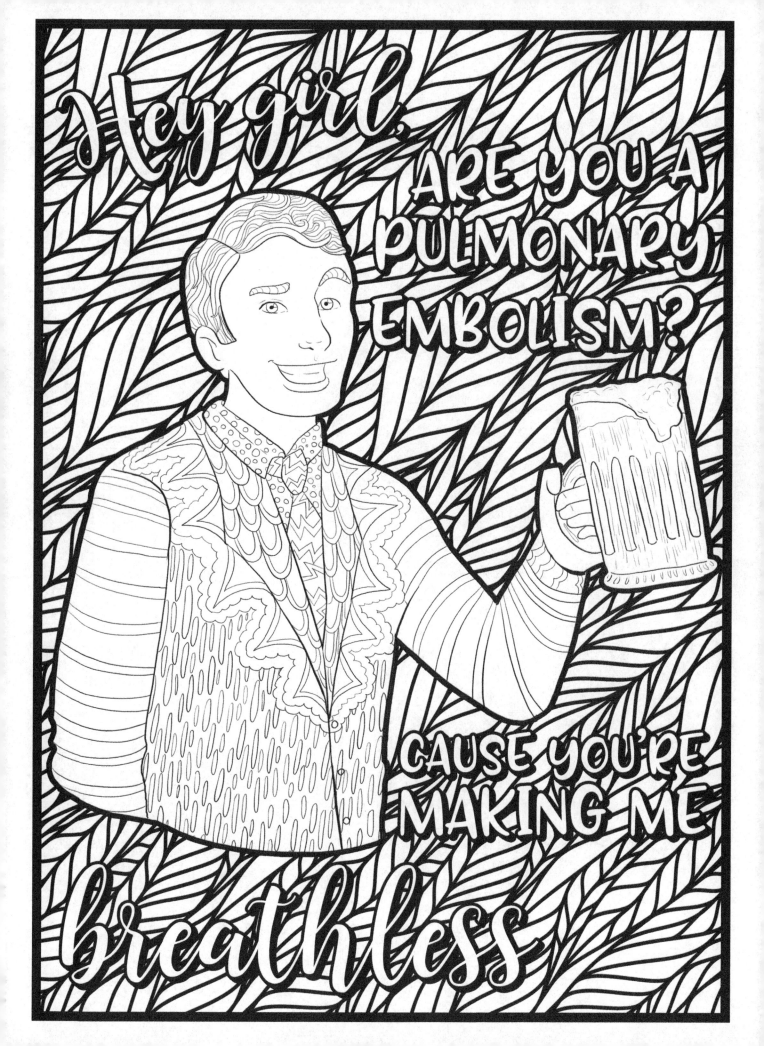

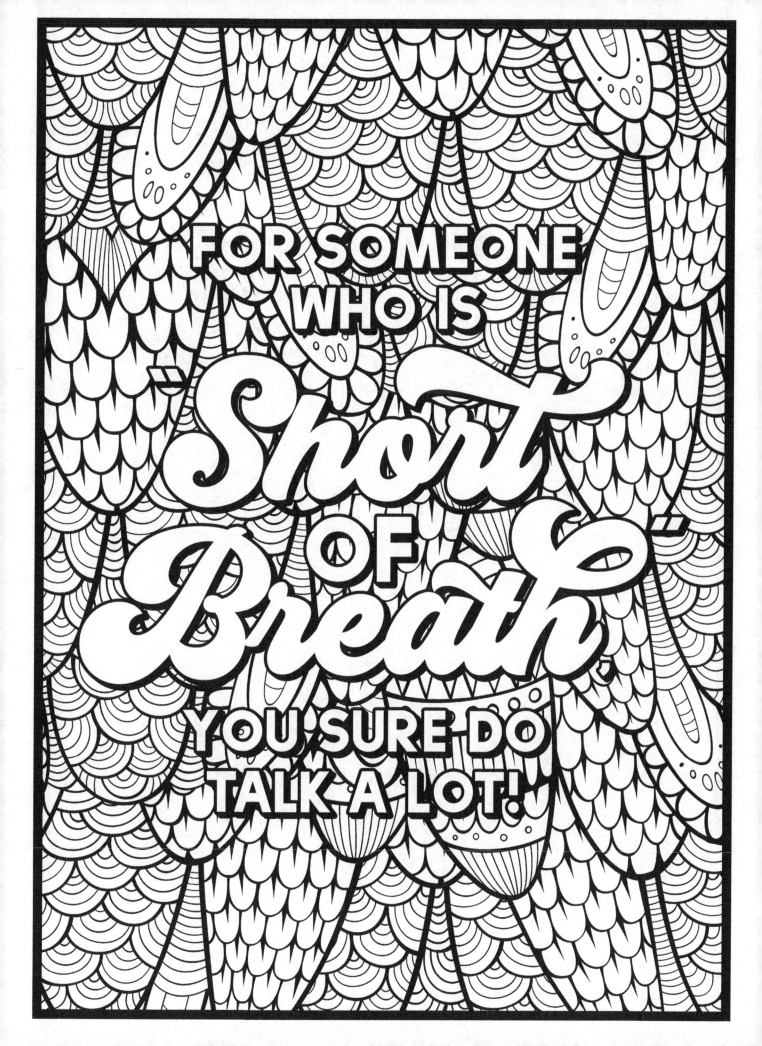

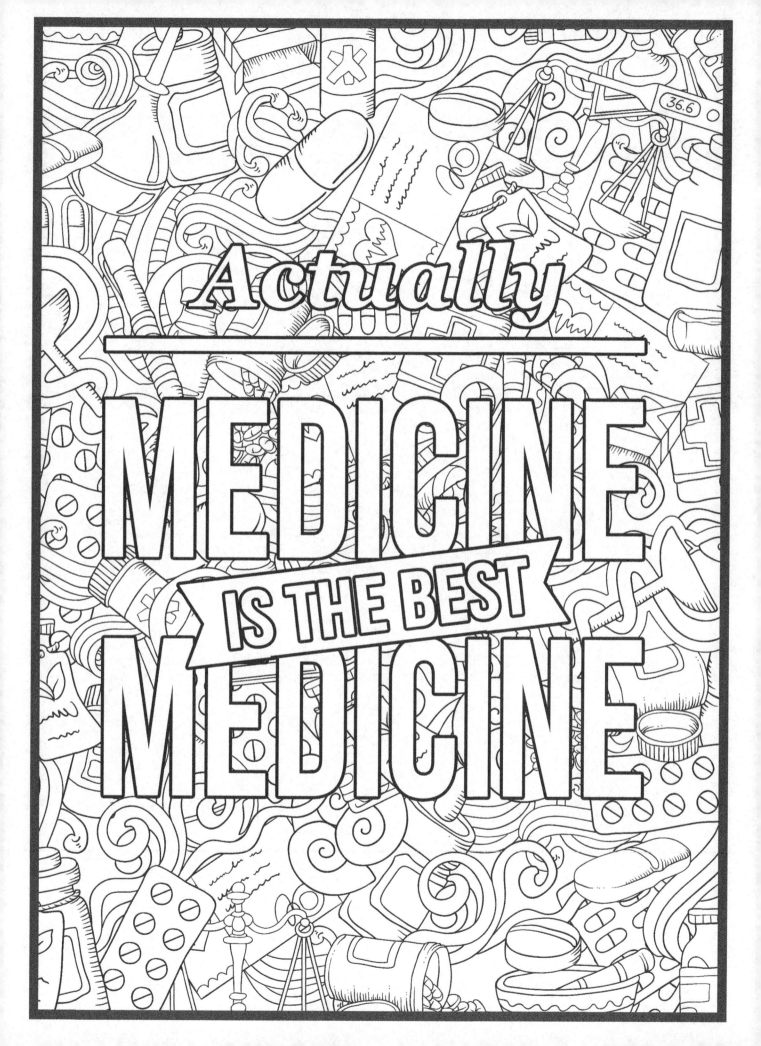

SORRY, BUT YOUR PASSWORD MUST CONTAIN A SYMBOL. A NUMBER. AN UPPERCASE LETTER. A HIEROGLYPH. A HAIKU. and THE BLOOD of a VIRGIN

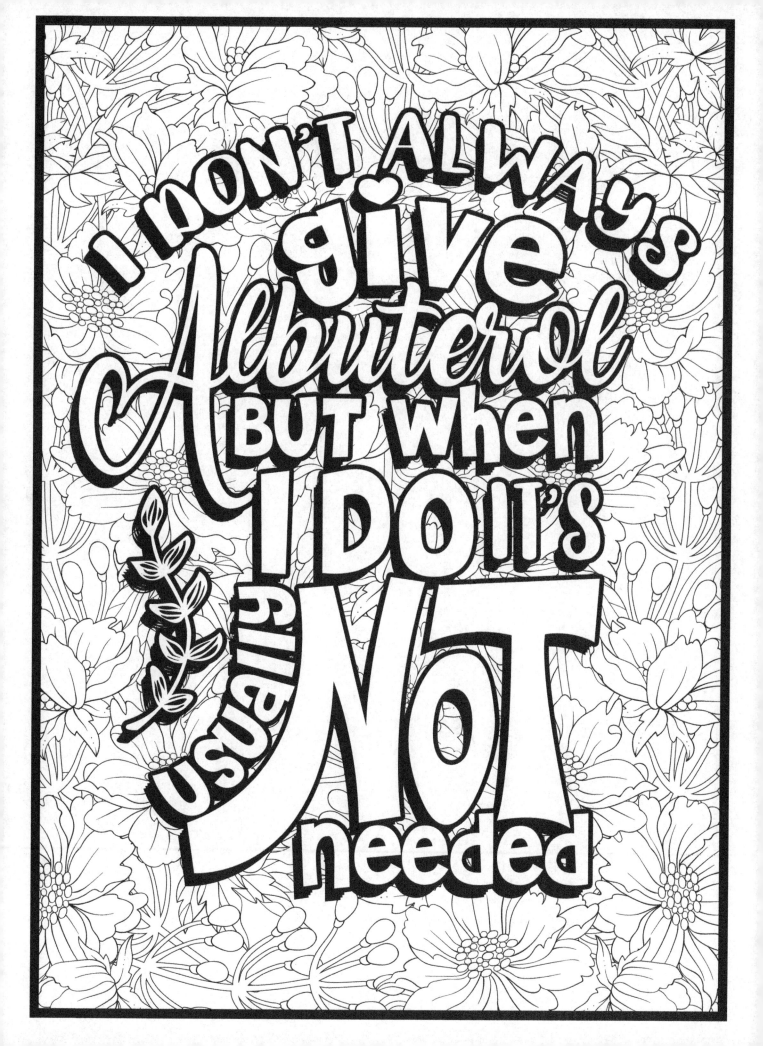

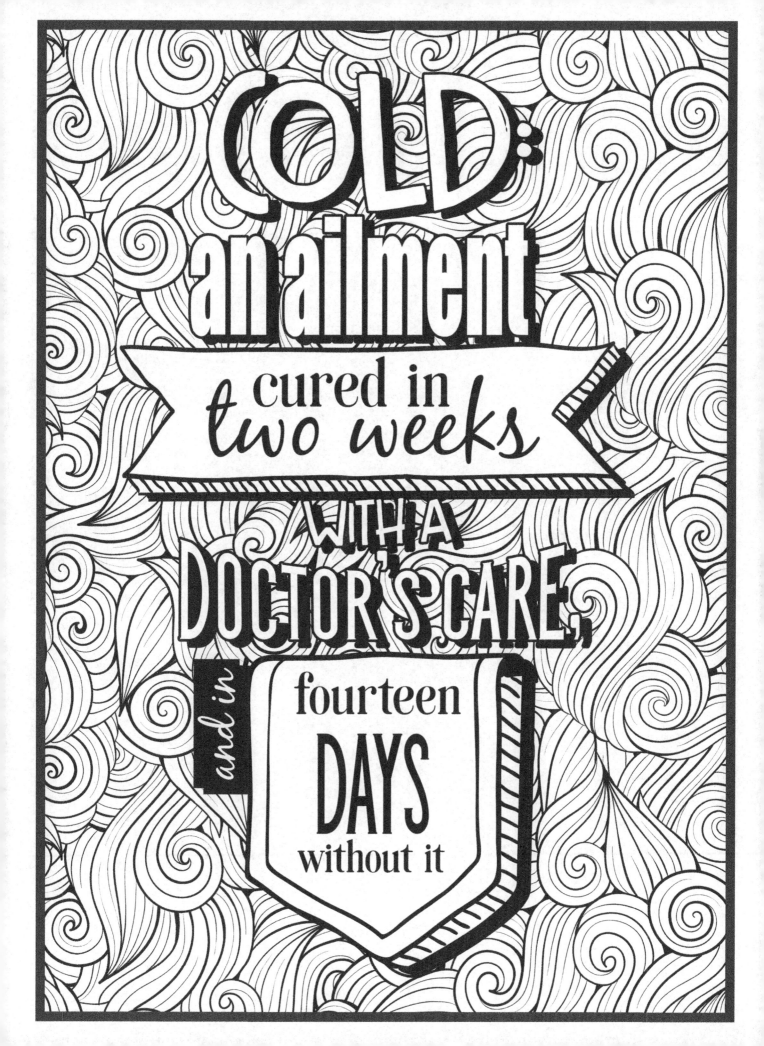

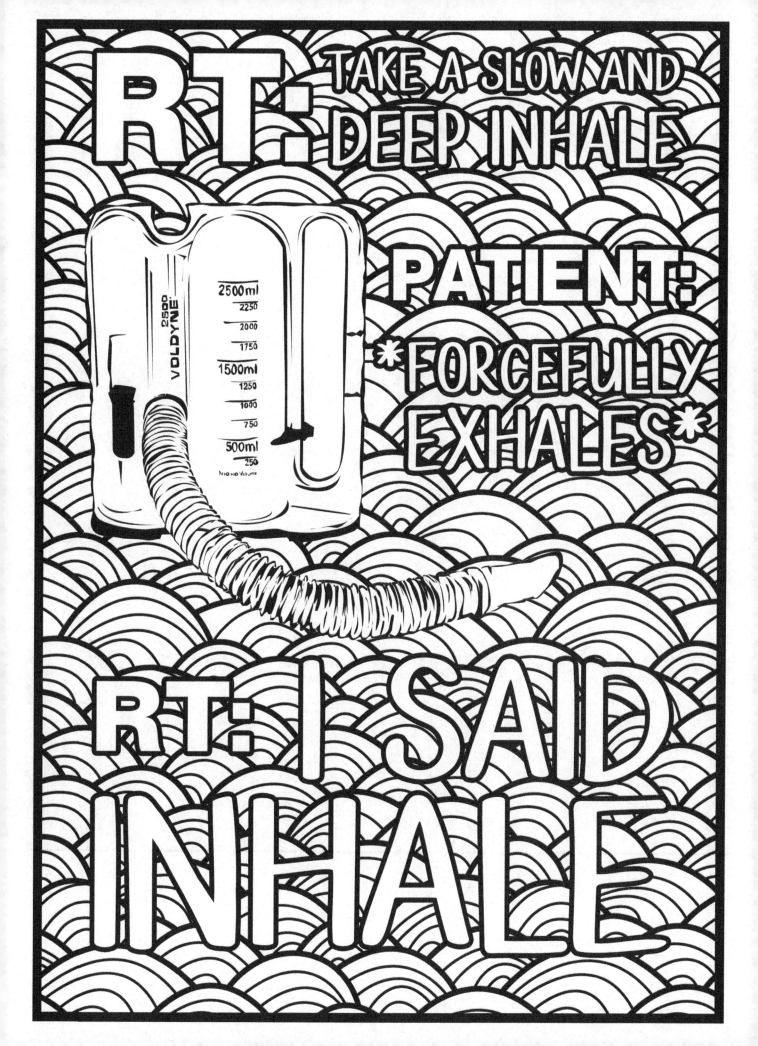

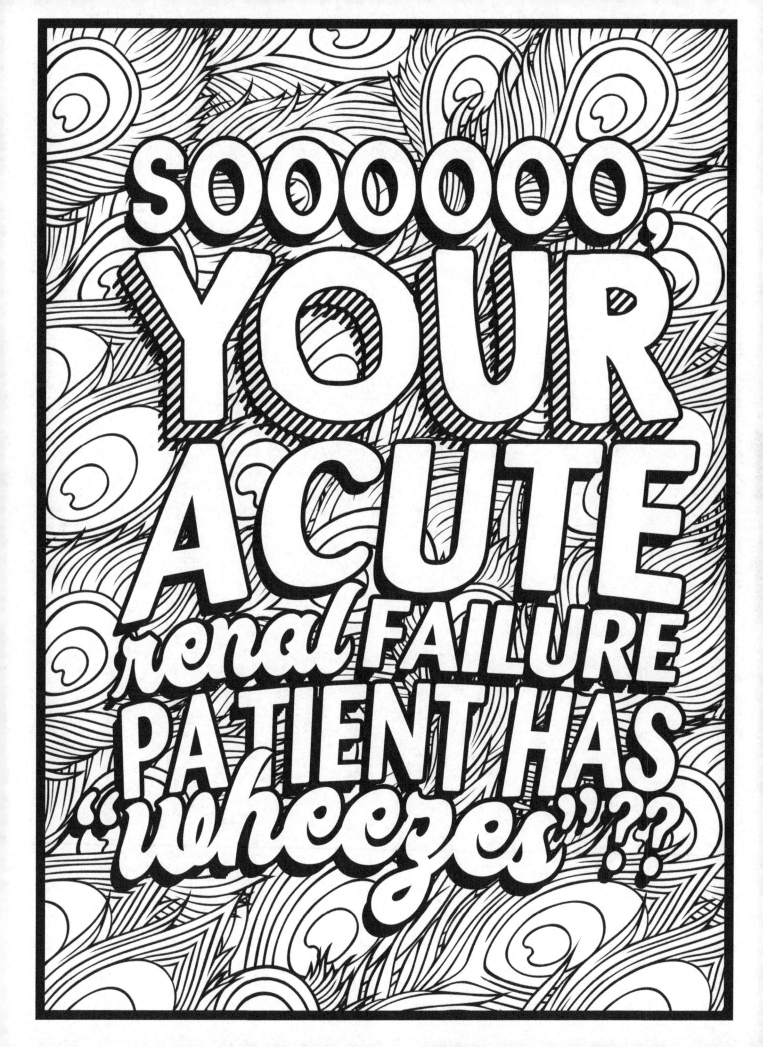

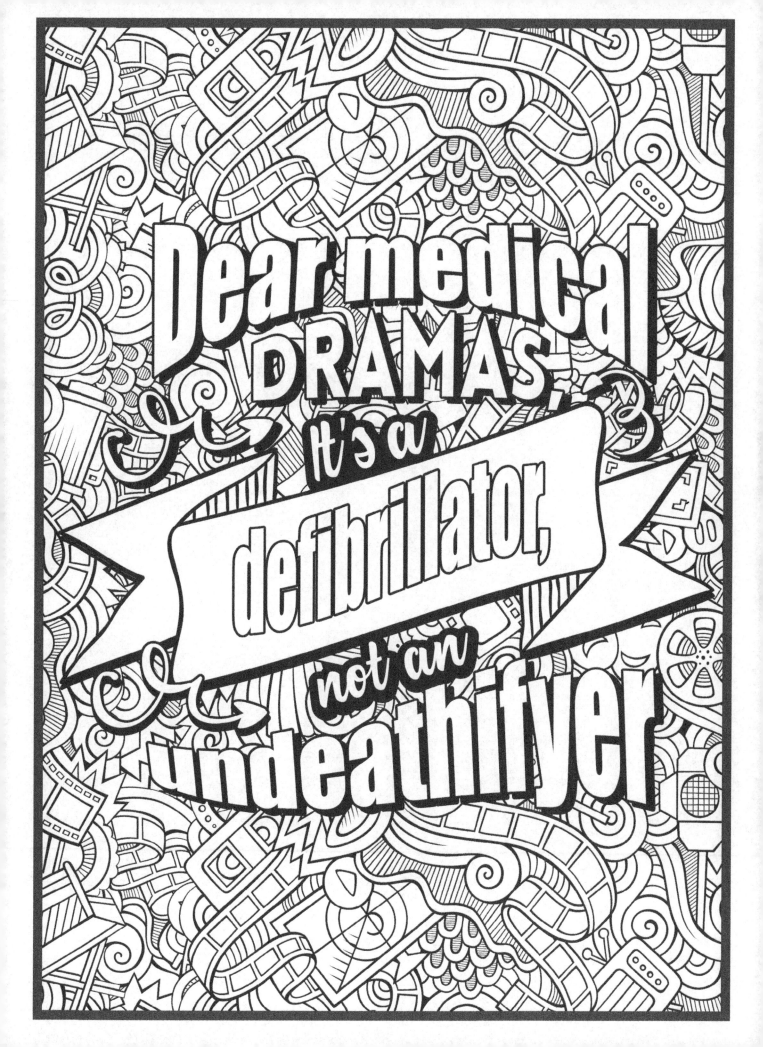

BEING A RT IS LIKE RIDING A BIKE.
EXCEPT THE BIKE IS ON FIRE AND YOU'RE ON FIRE
AND EVERYTHING IS ON FIRE BECAUSE YOU'RE IN
HELL

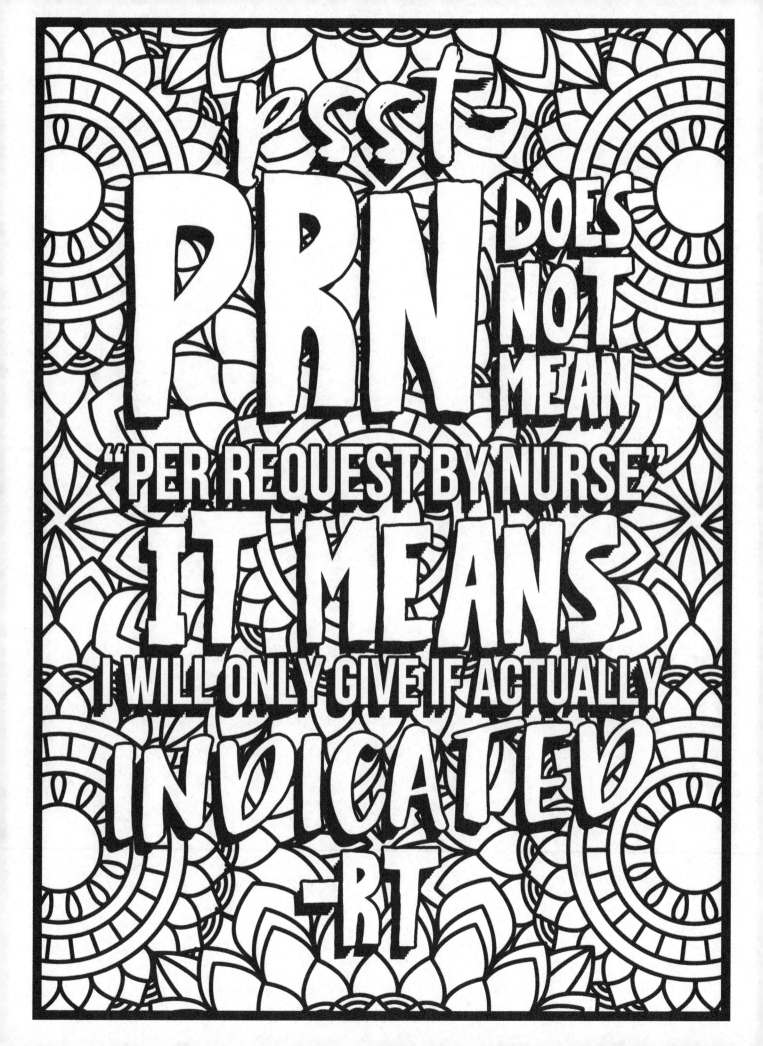

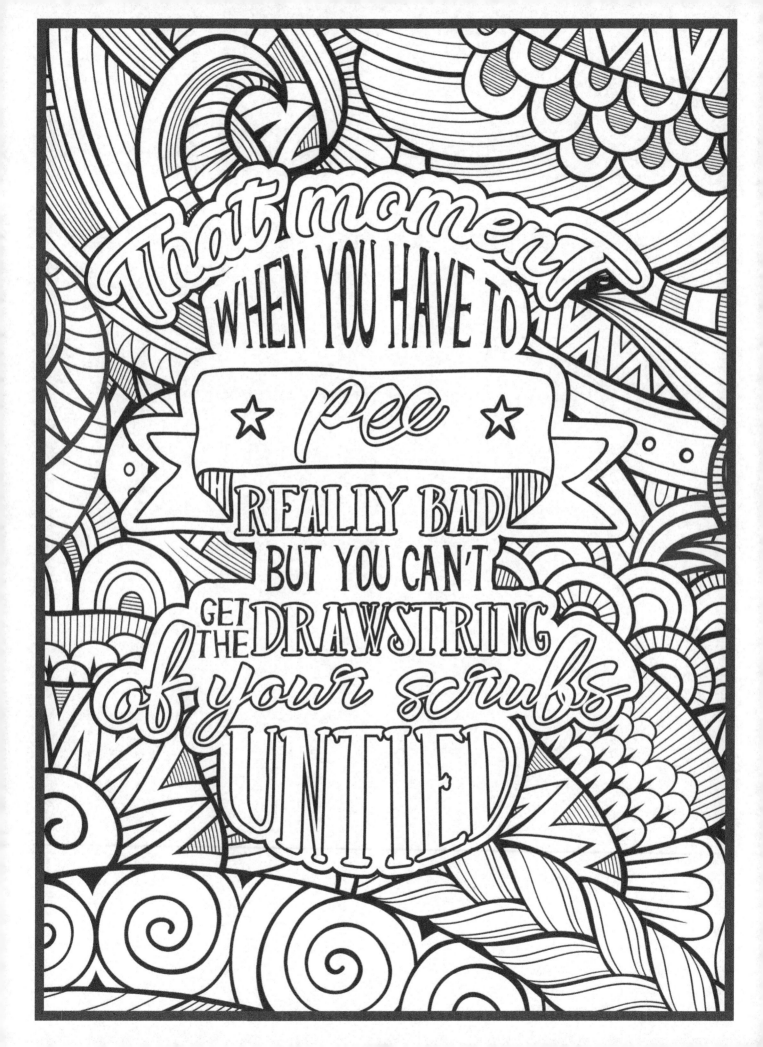

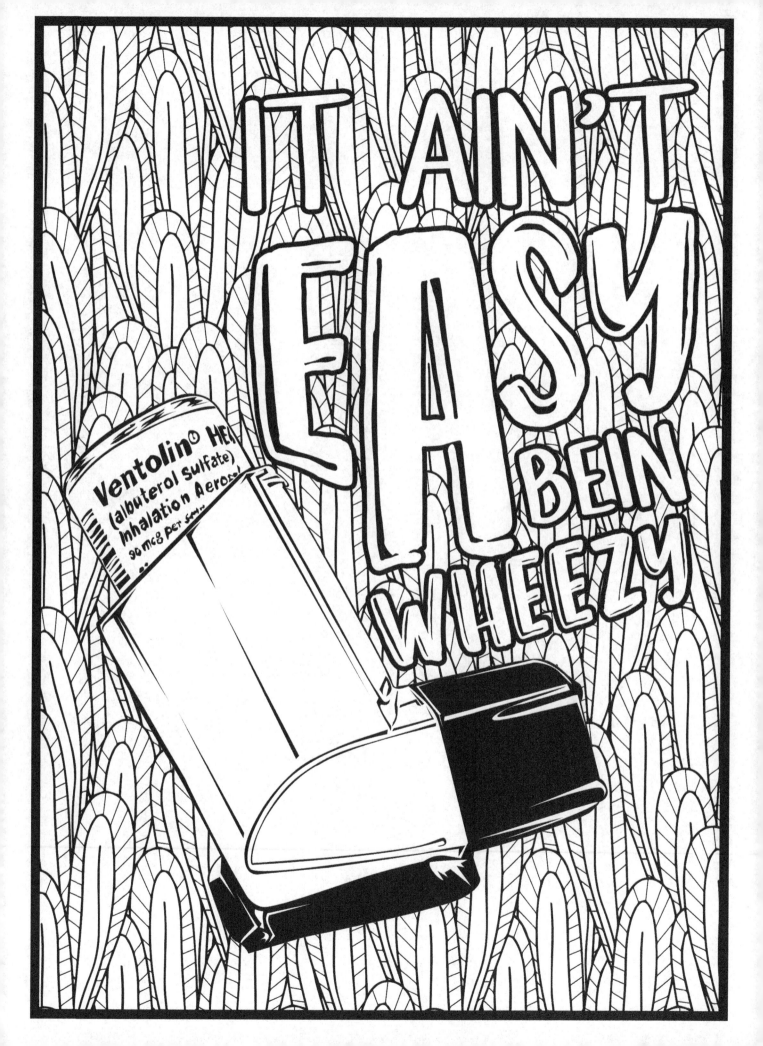

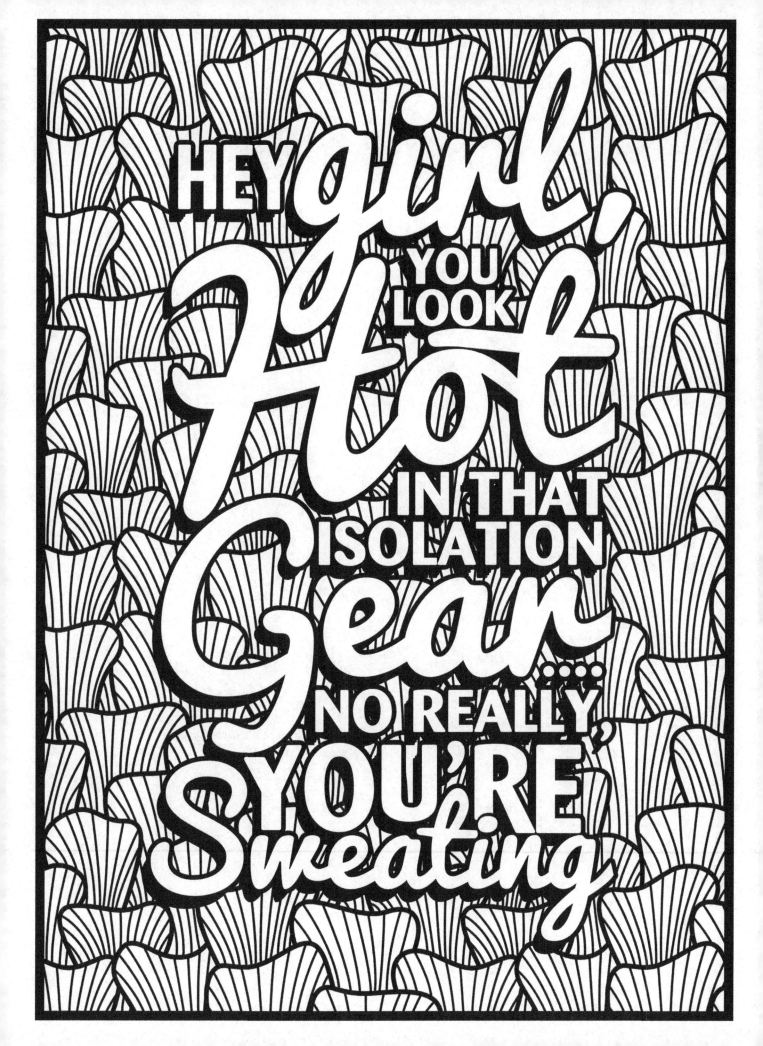

LIVIN' THE SCRUB LIFE

when i find out my patient is on isolation precautions after i've already BEEN in the Room a million times

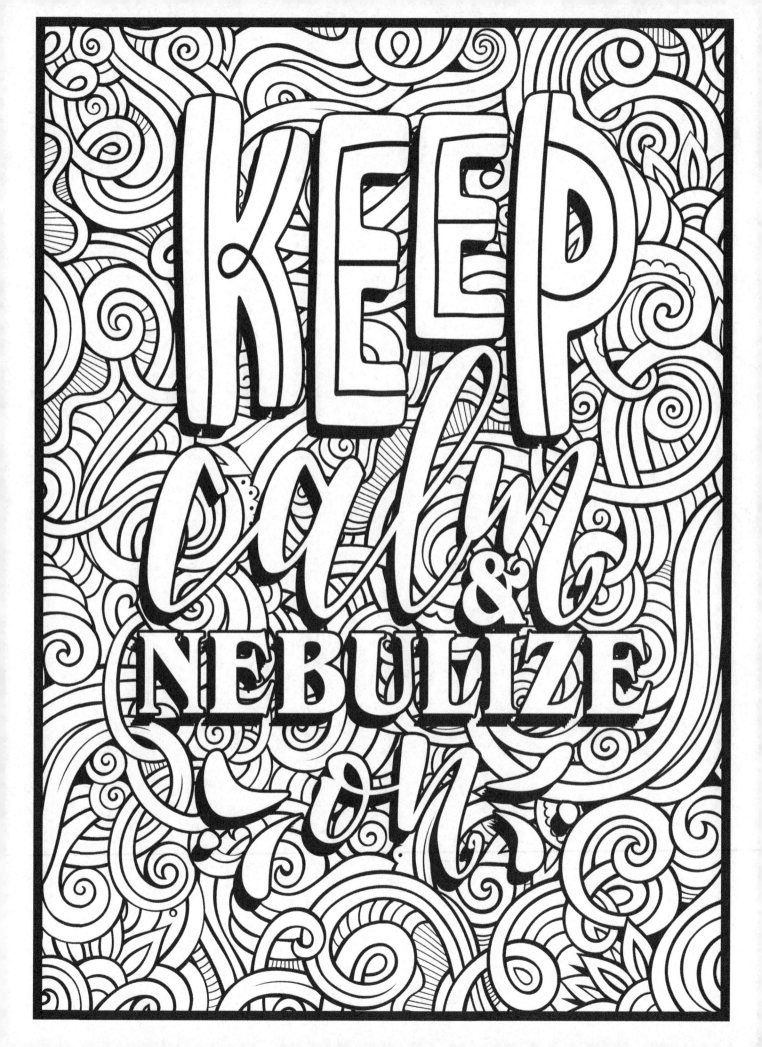

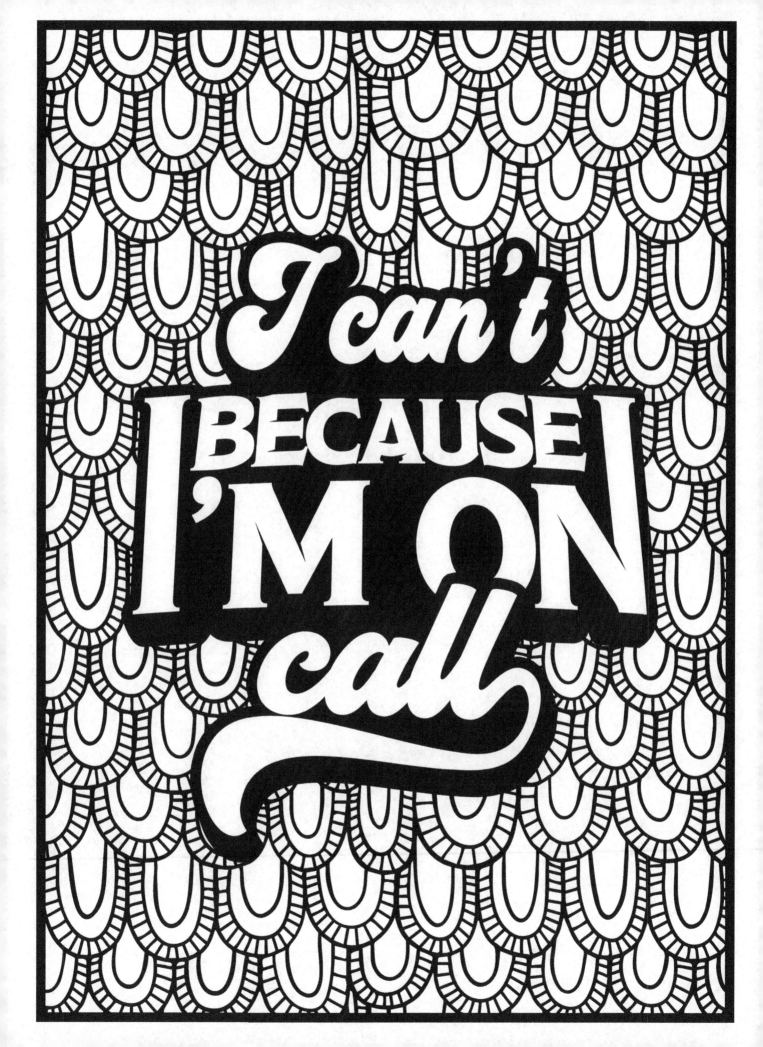

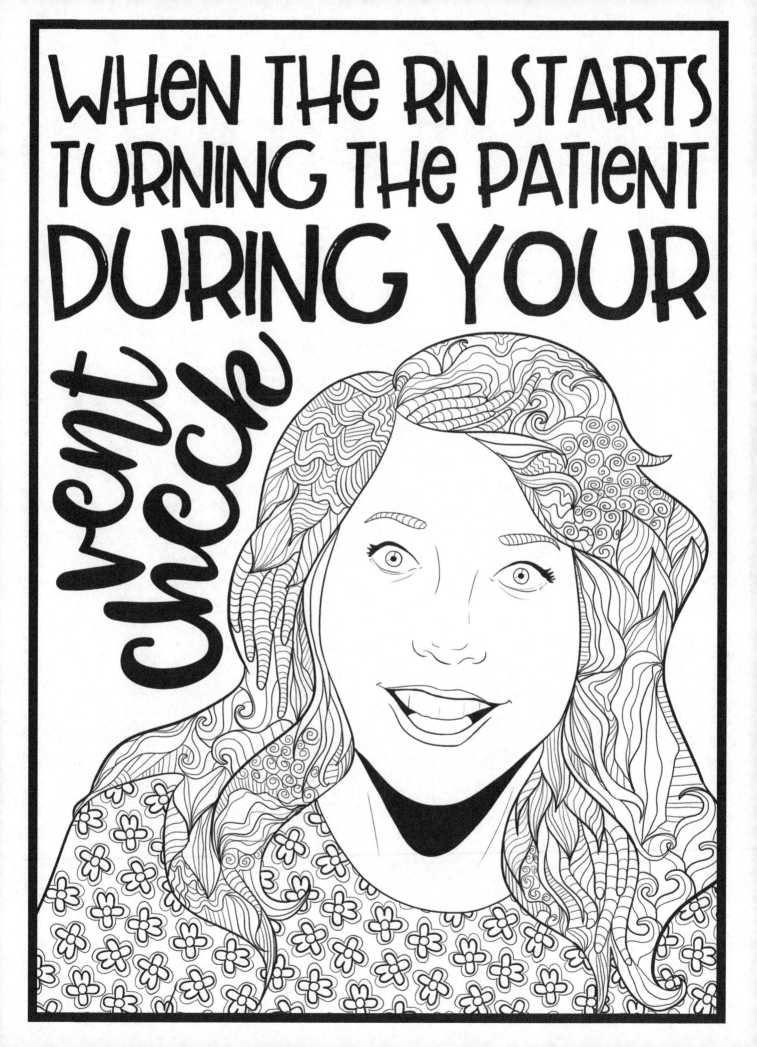

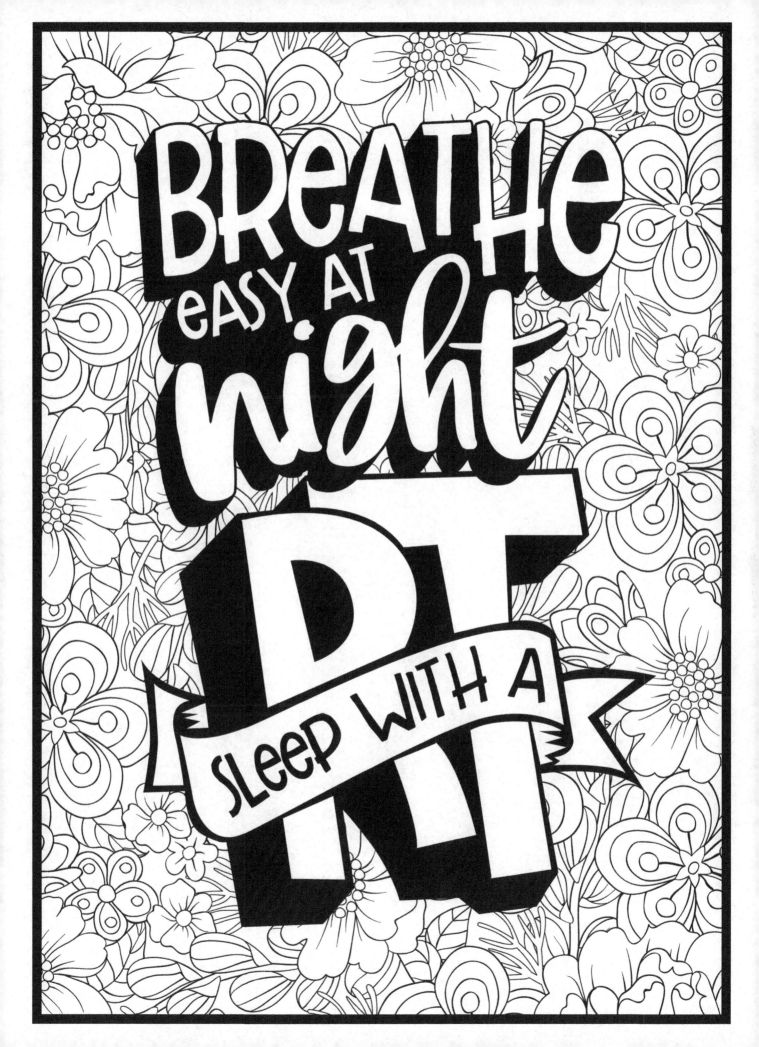

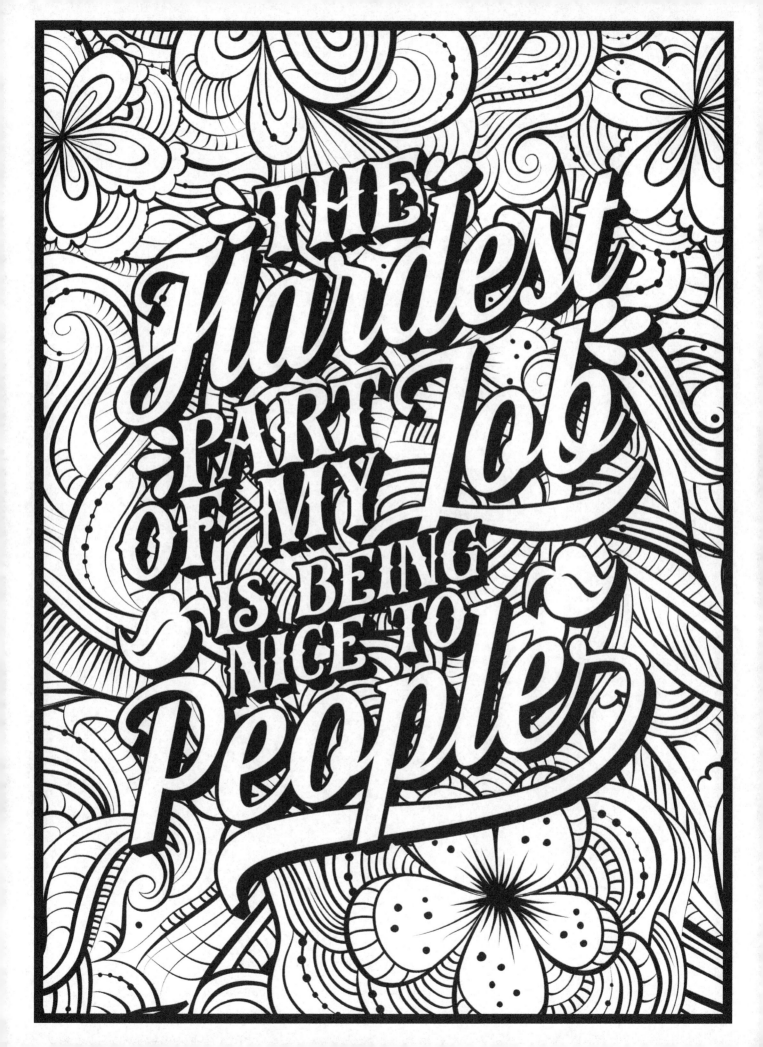

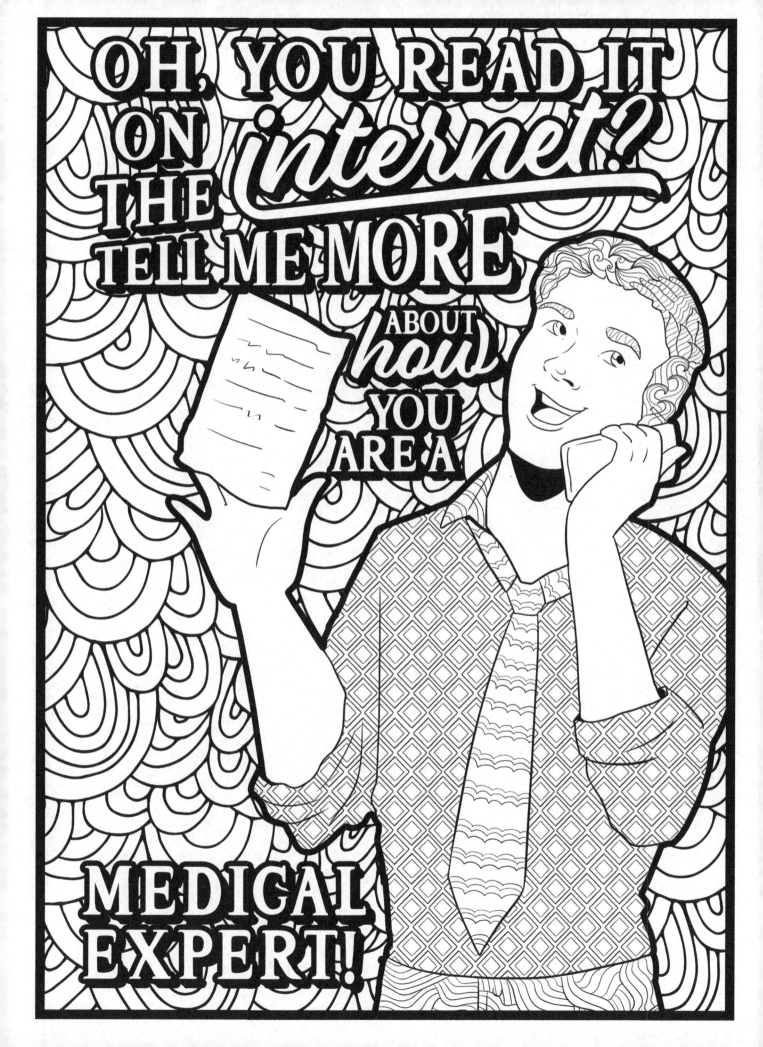

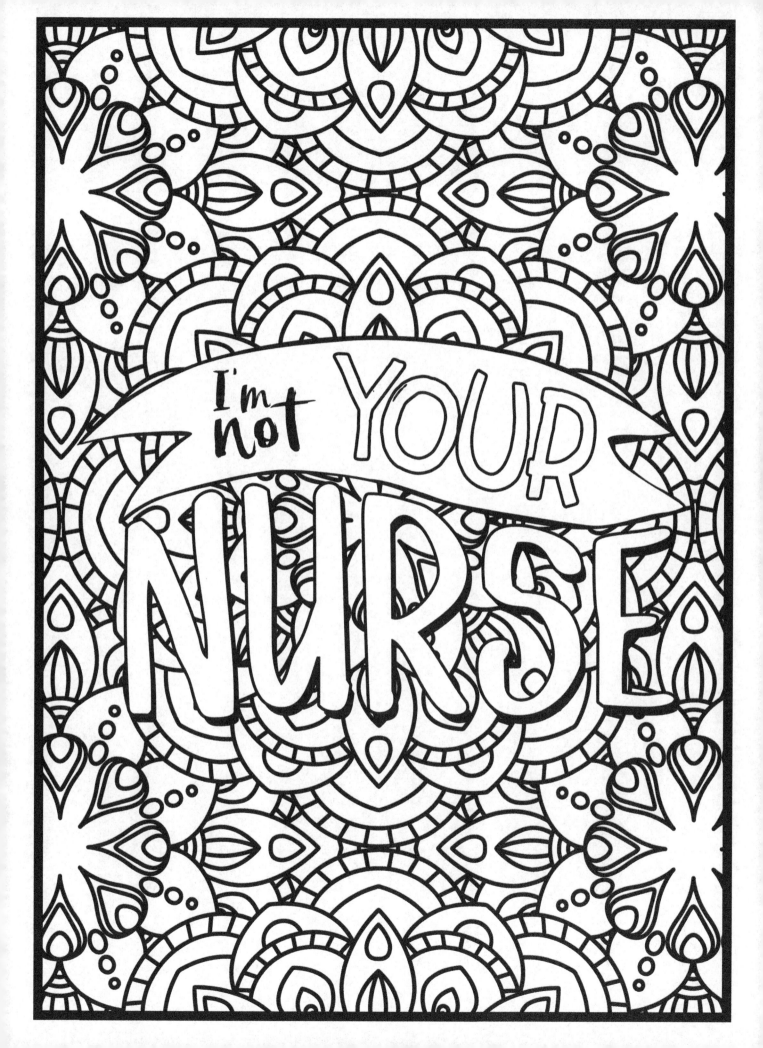

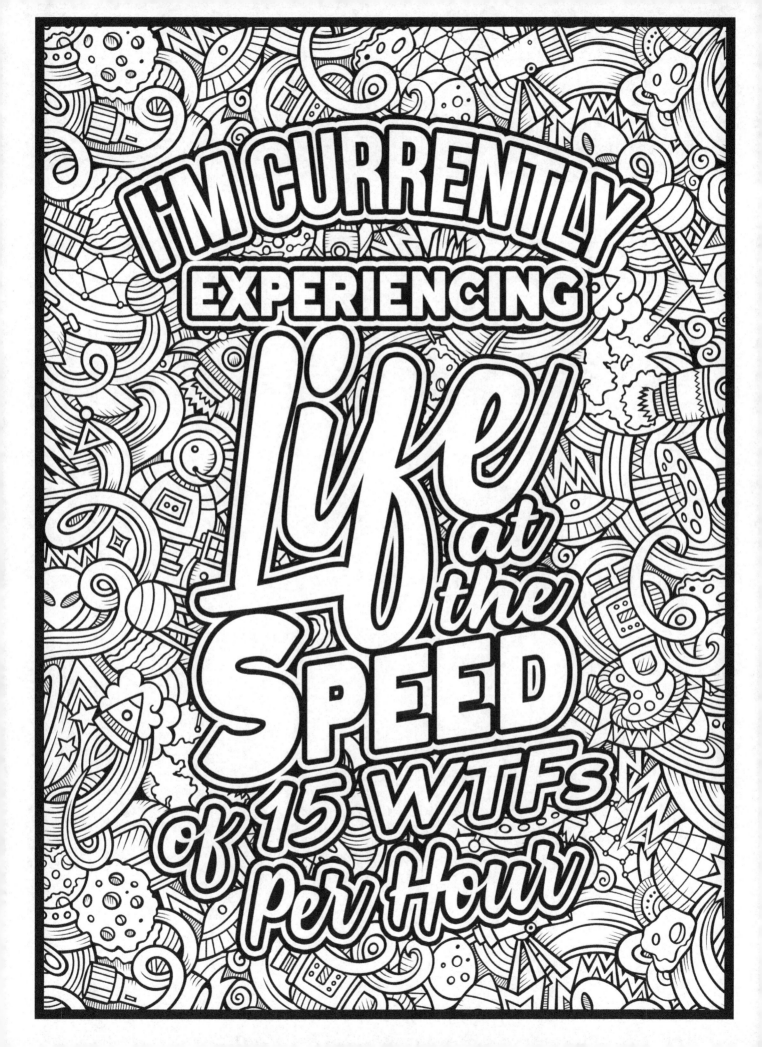

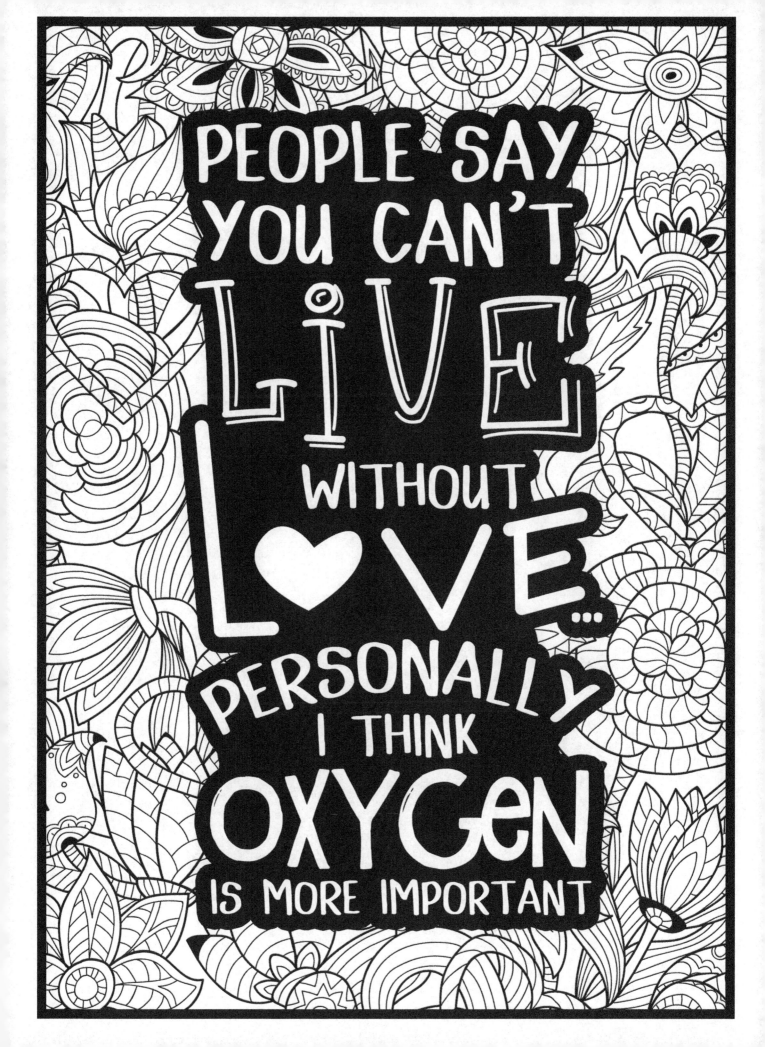

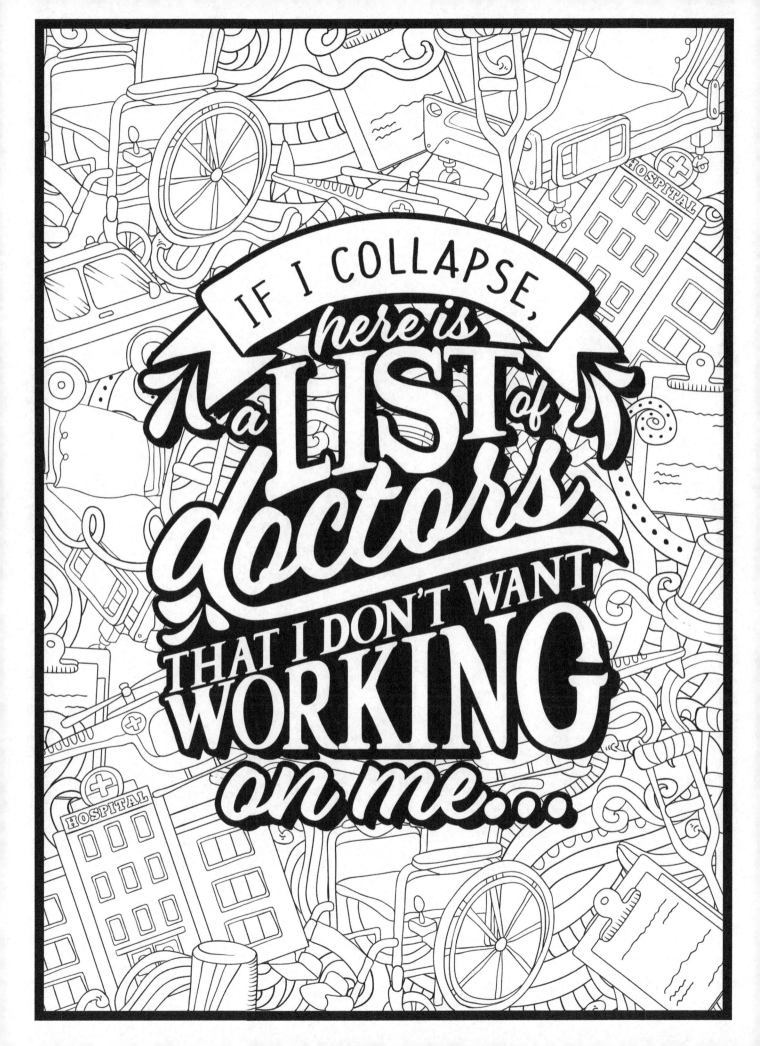

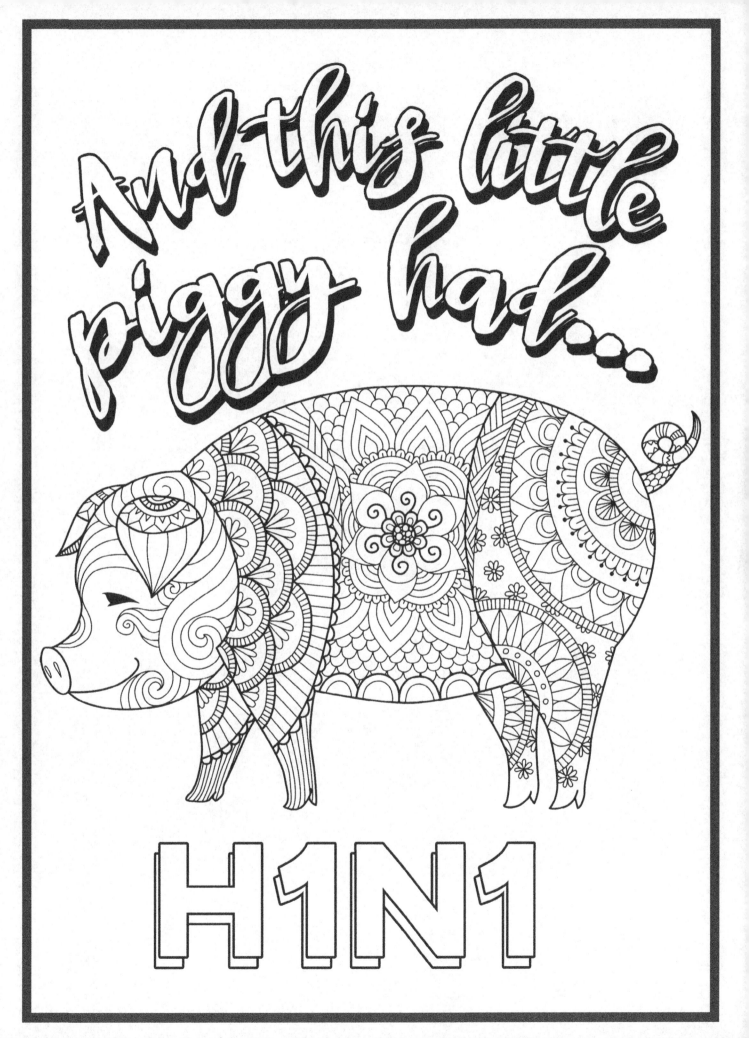

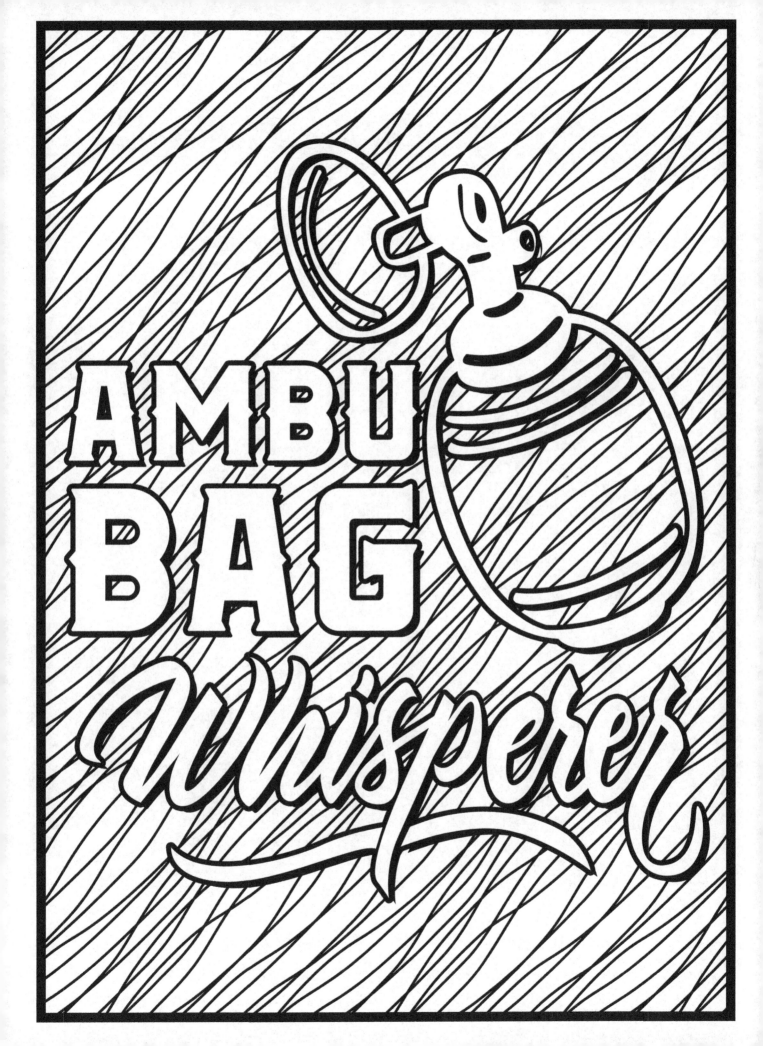

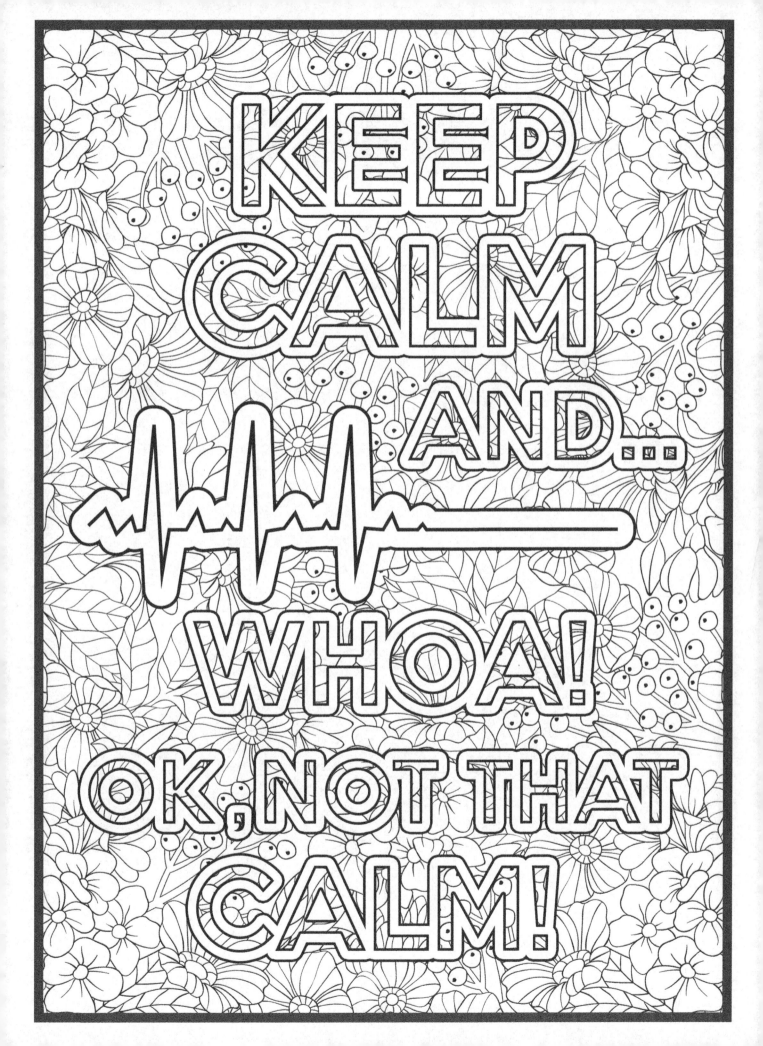

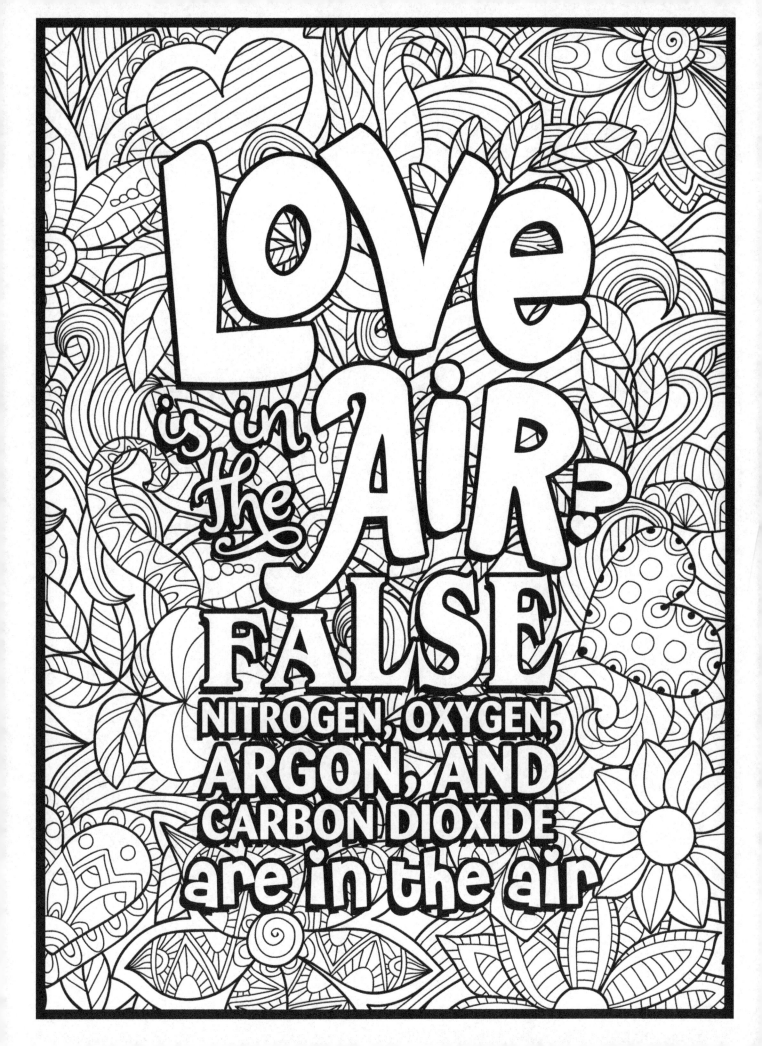

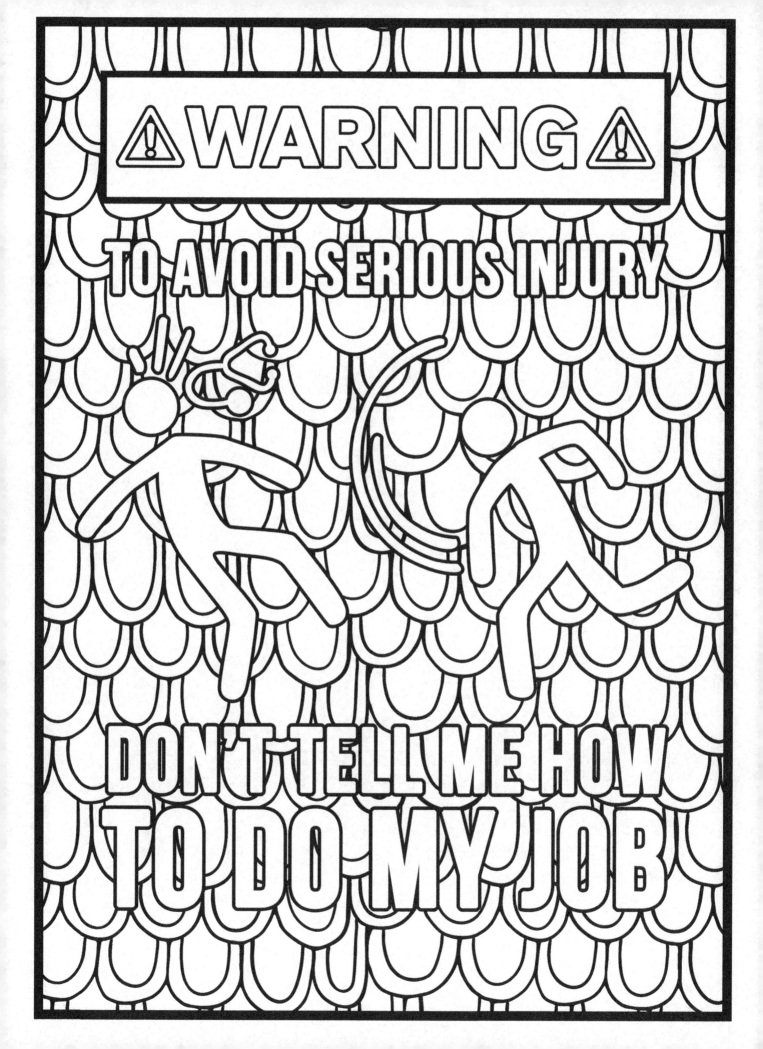

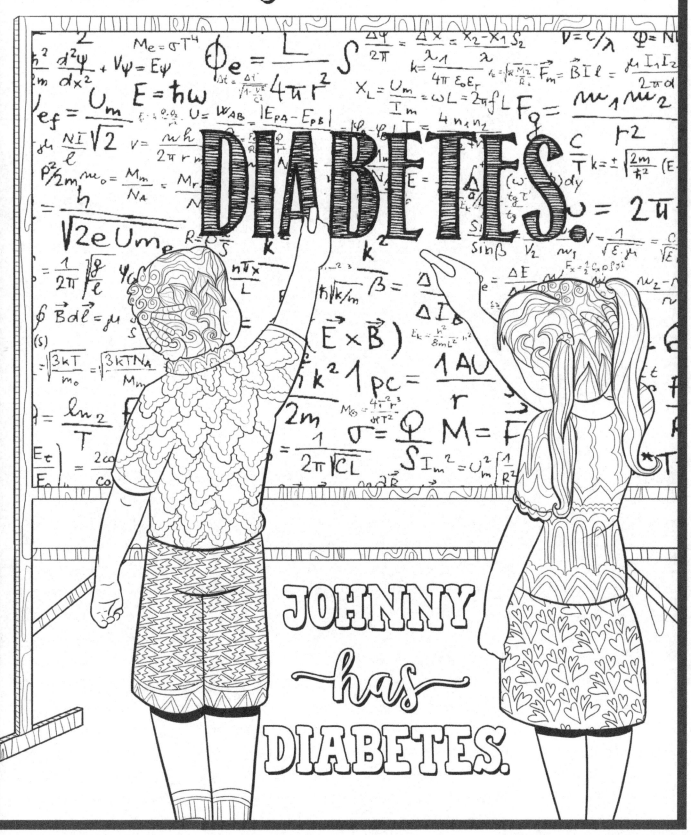

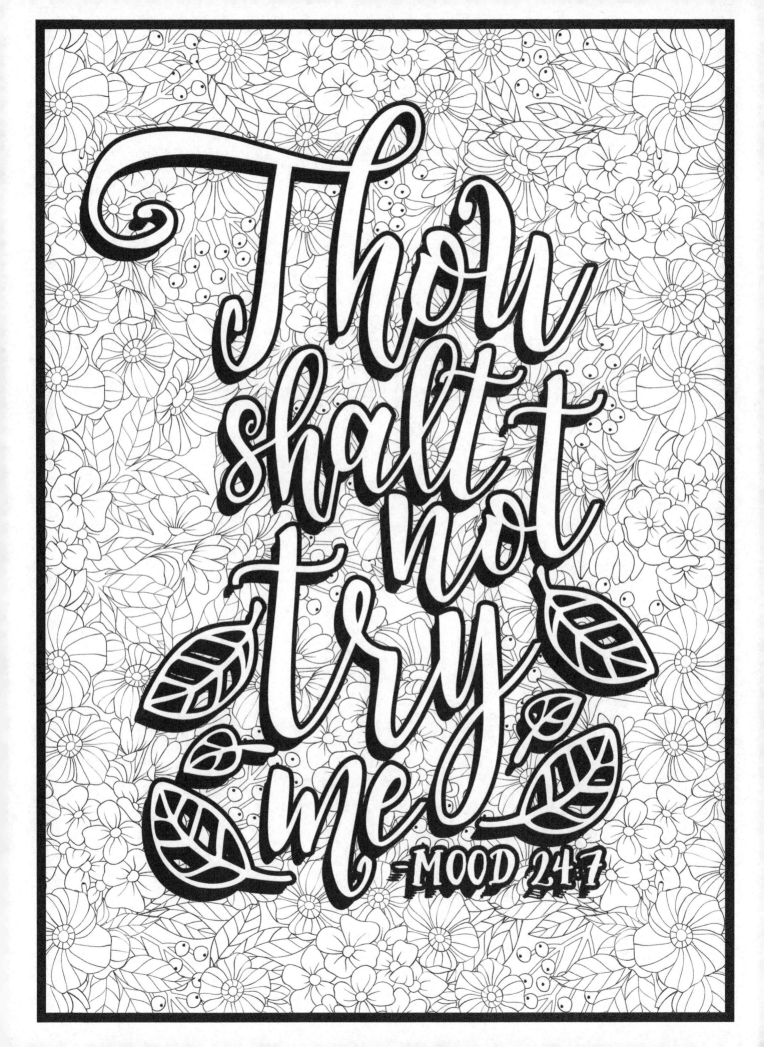

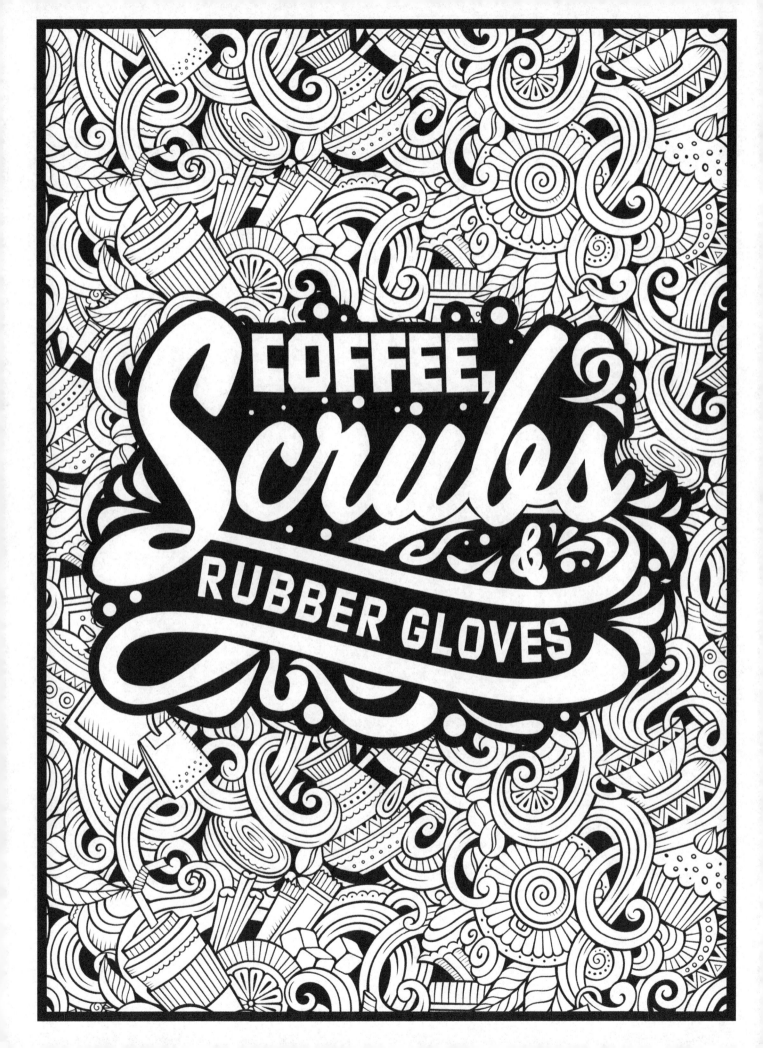

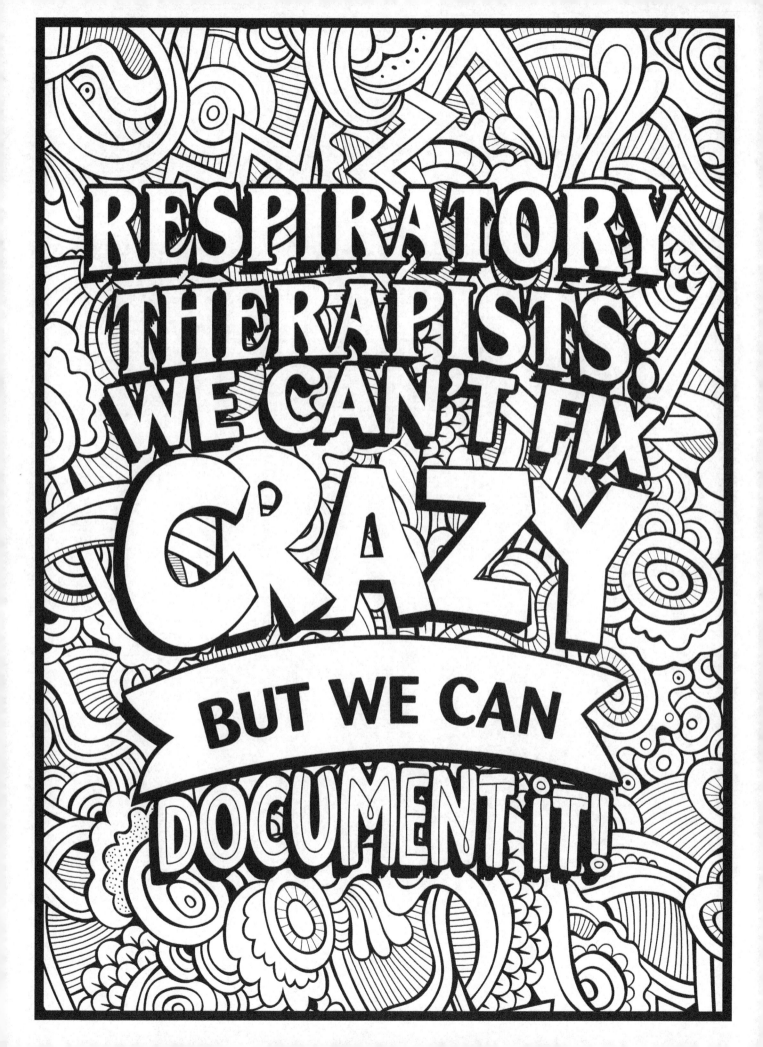

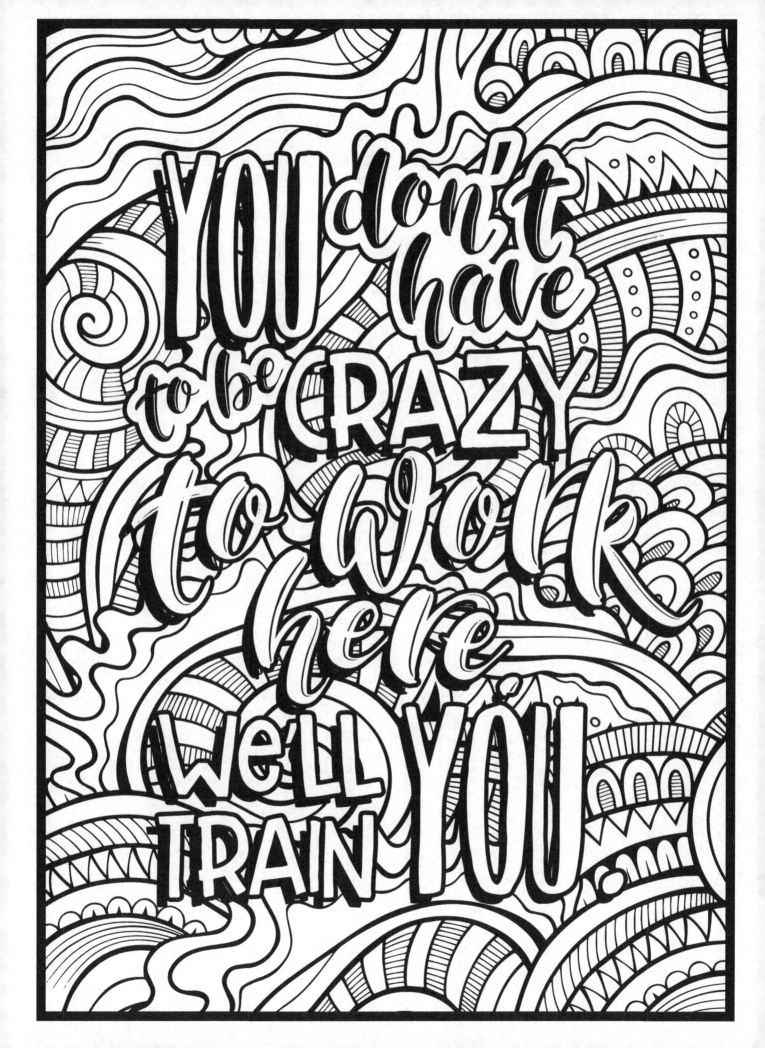

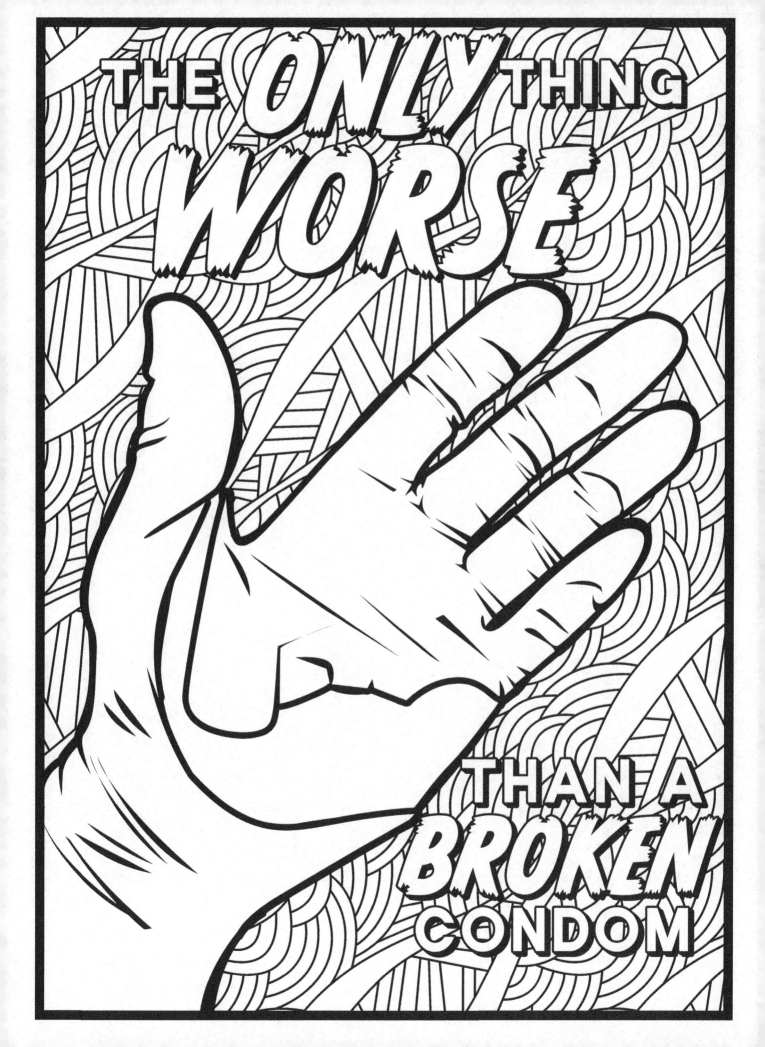

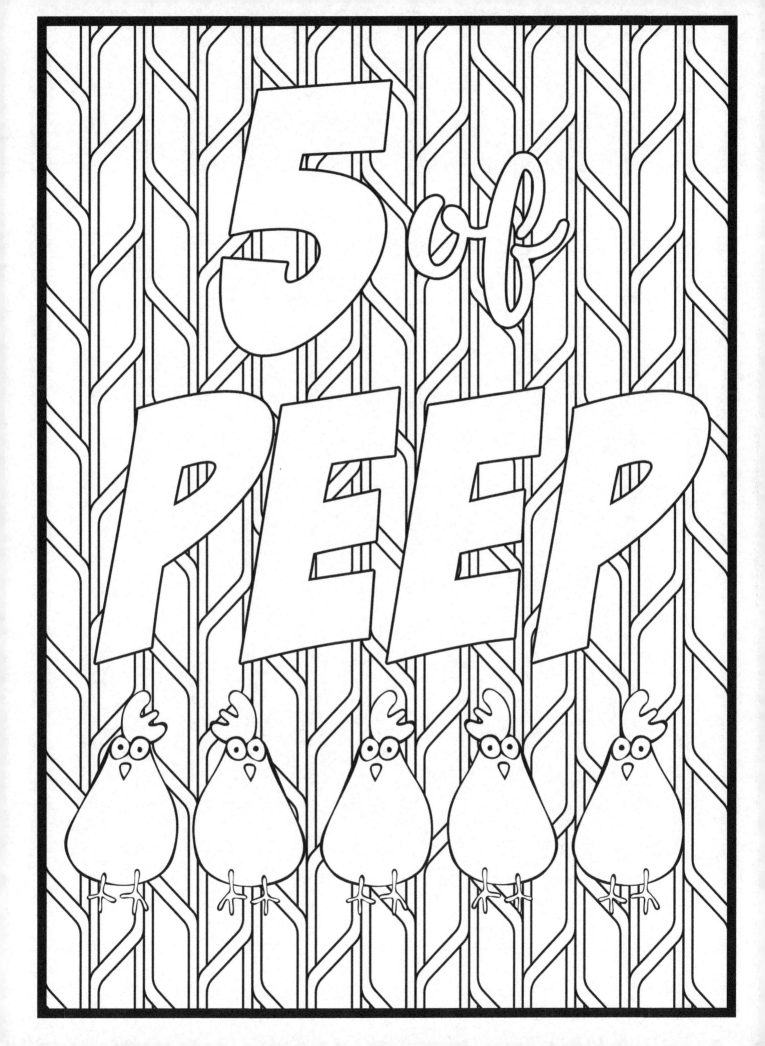

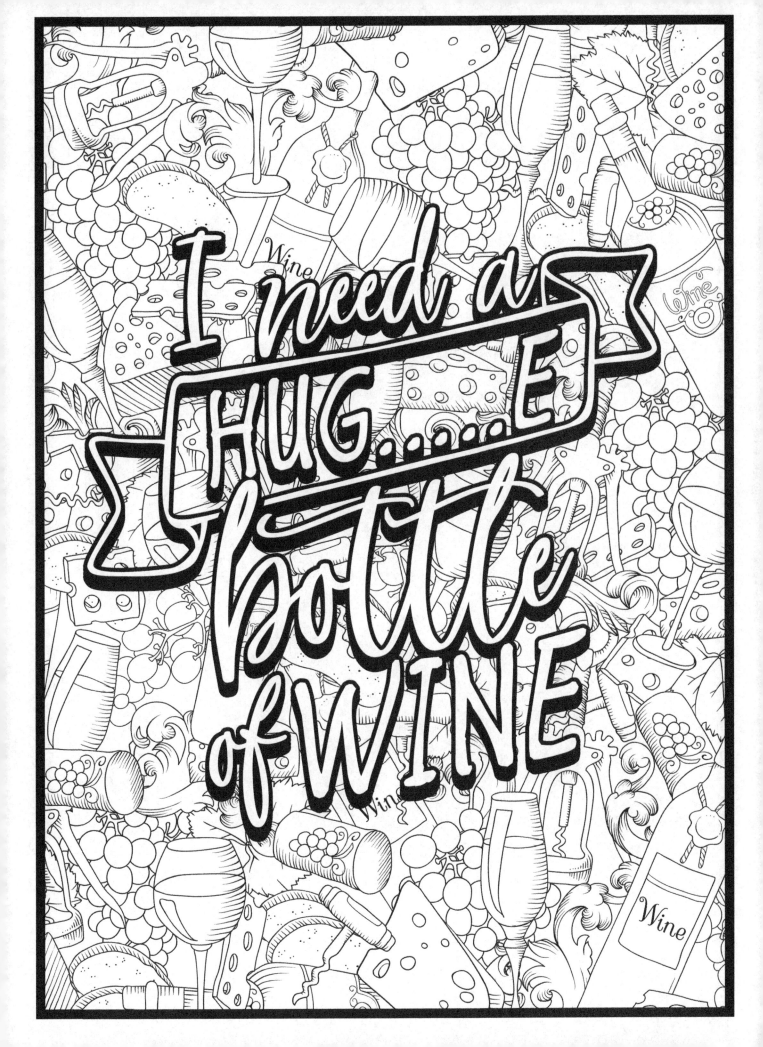

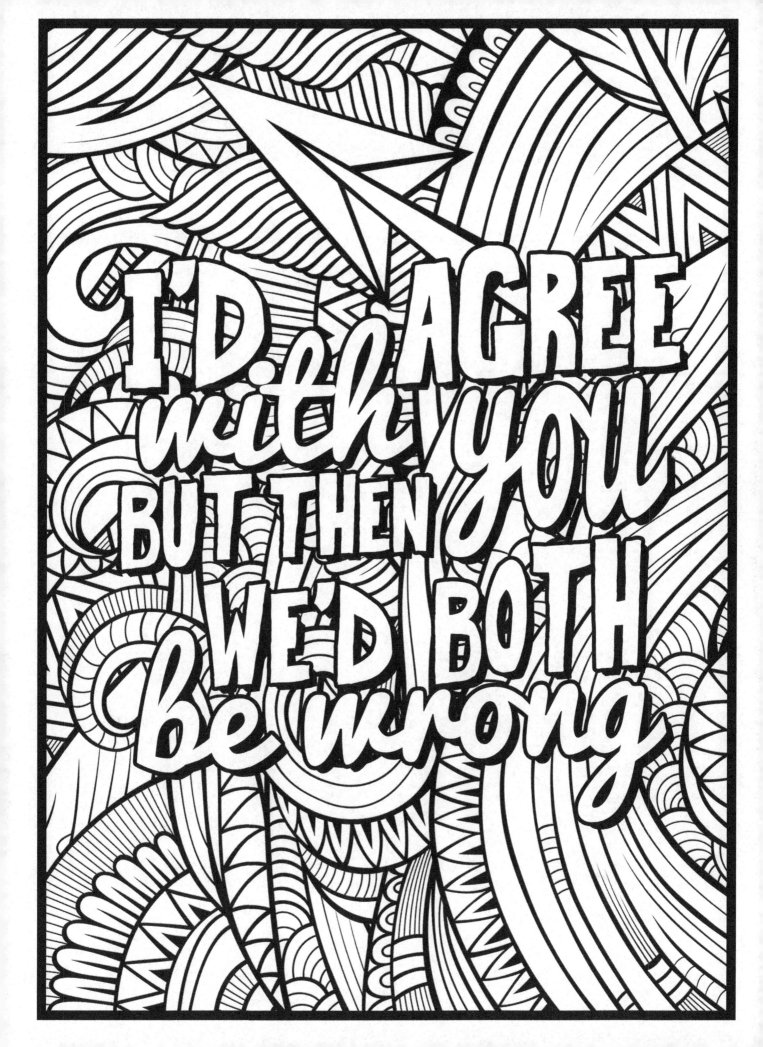

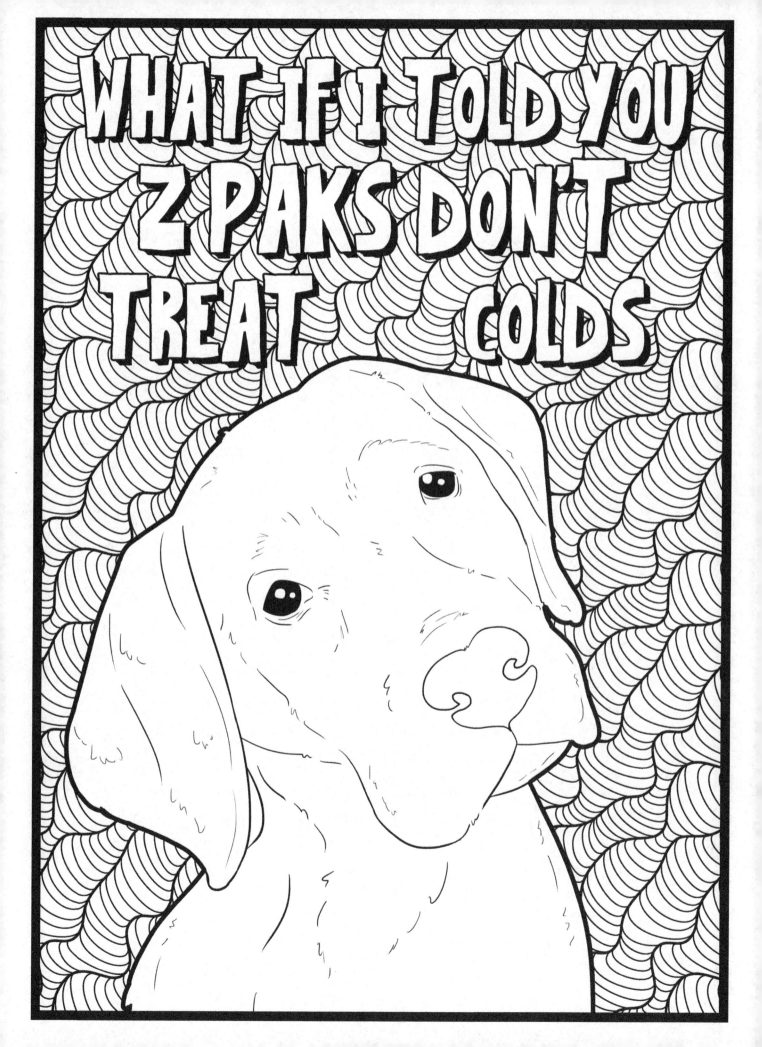

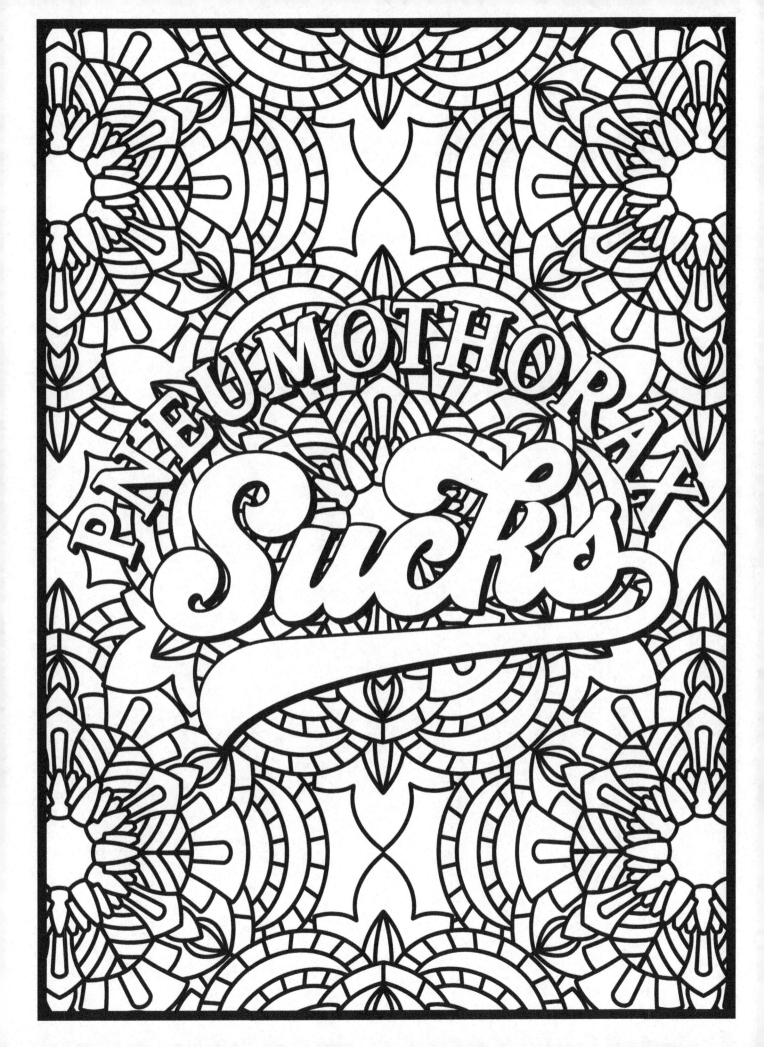

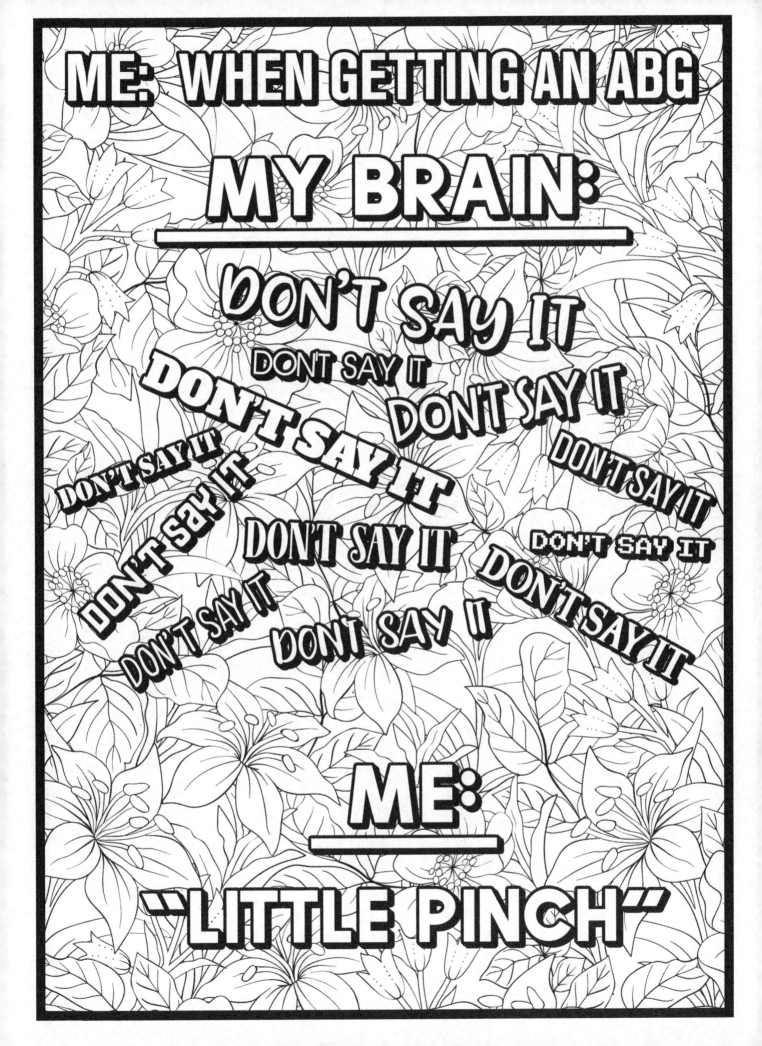

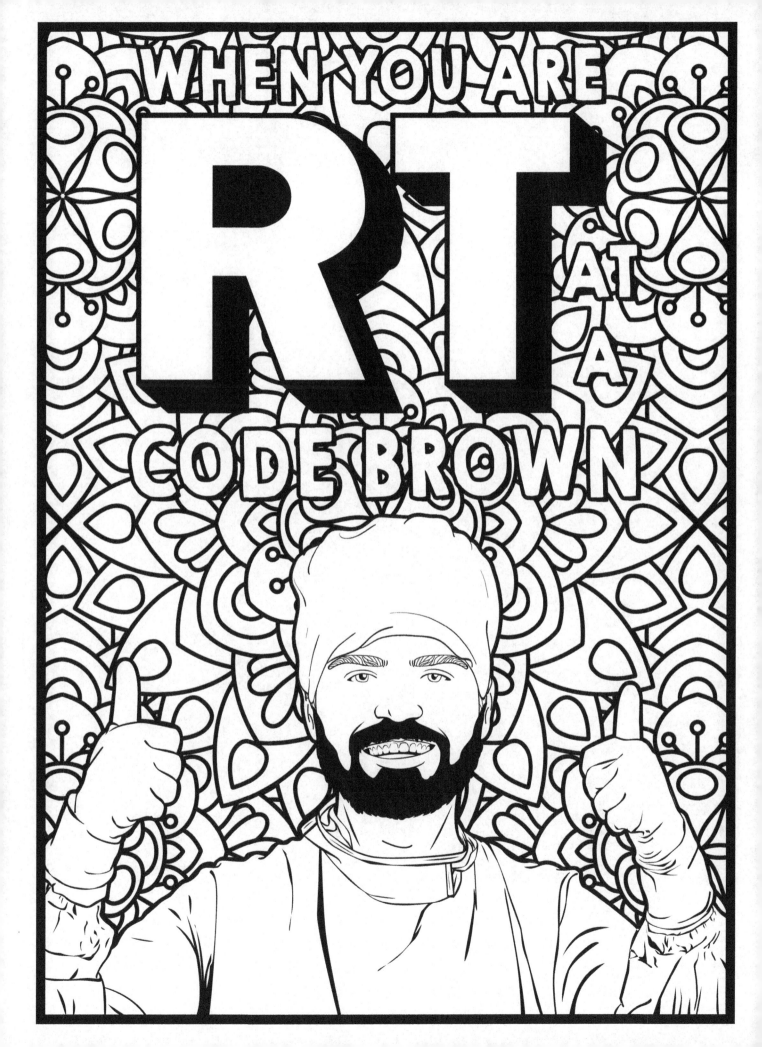

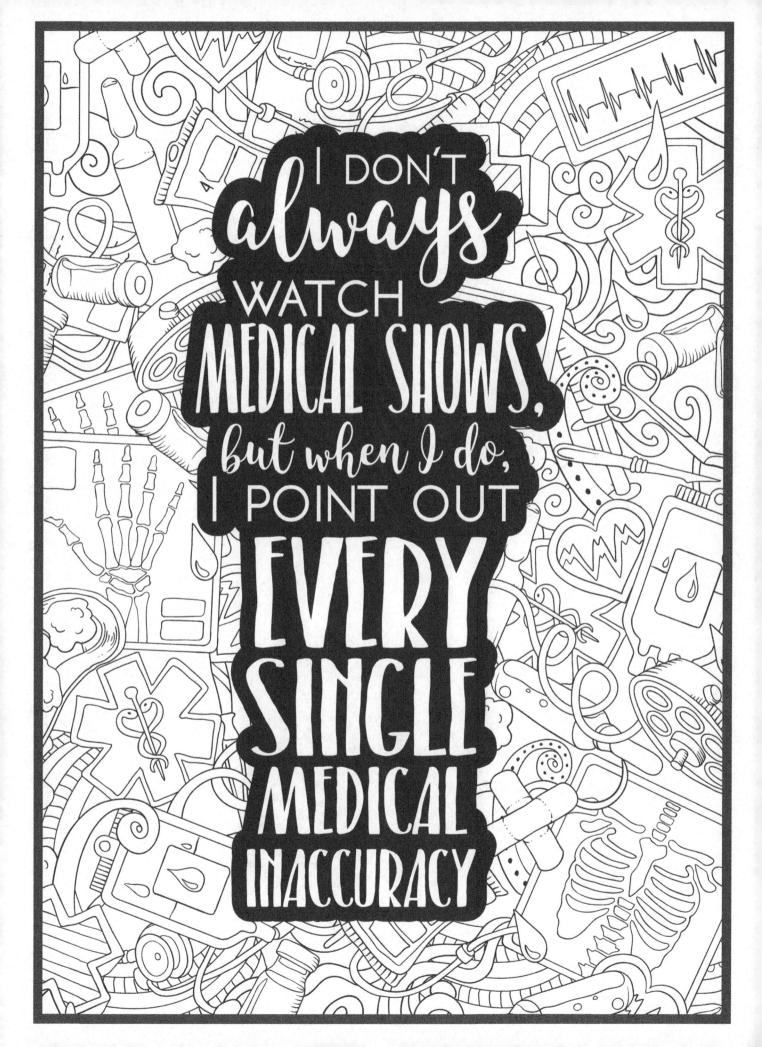

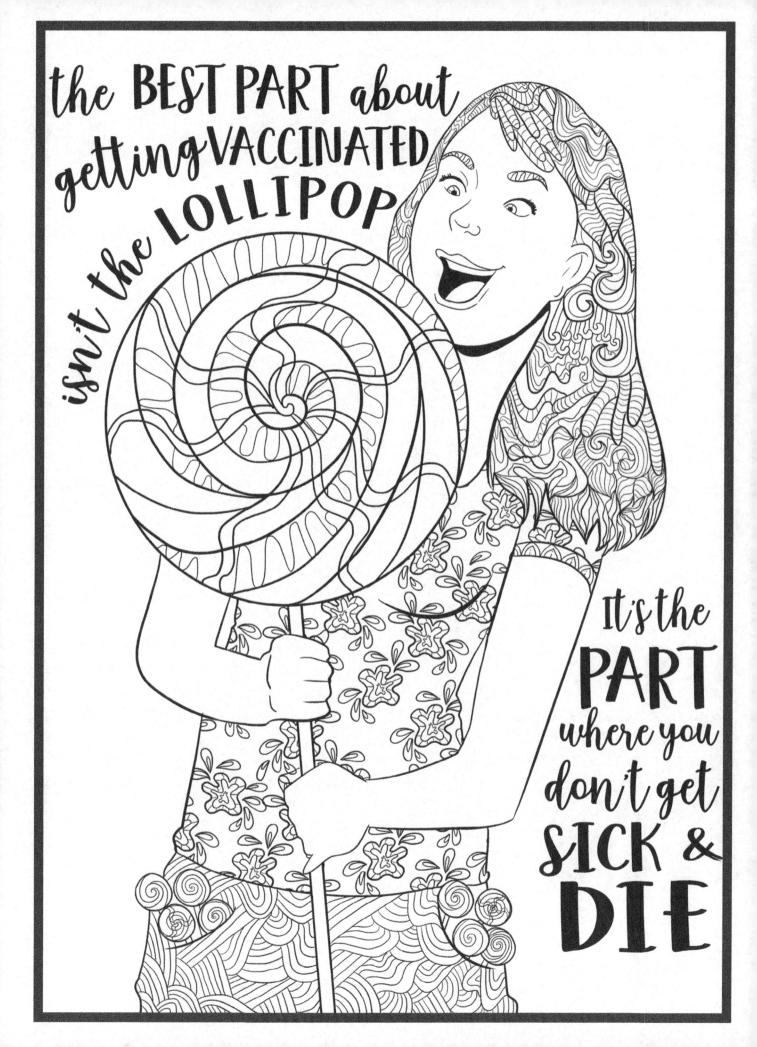

FREEBIE!

JOIN OUR VIP NEWSLETTER AND RECEIVE A FREE DIGITAL DOWNLOAD OF A PRINTABLE PDF <u>ACTIVITY BOOK FOR ADULTS</u> FEATURING INSPIRATIONAL QUOTE COLORING PAGES, MANDALAS, WORD SEARCHES, AND MAZES FOR ADULTS.

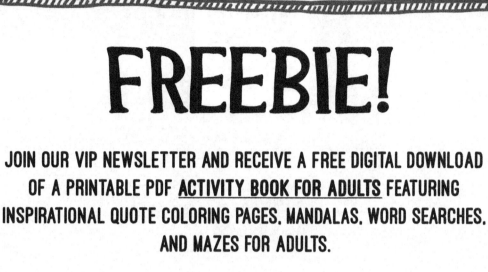

SIGN UP HERE

http://freebies.papeteriebleu.com/FRB3

@papeteriebleu

Papeterie Bleu

Shop our other books at
www.pbleu.com

Wholesale distribution through Ingram Content Group
www.ingramcontent.com/publishers/distribution/wholesale

For questions and customer service, email us at
support@pbleu.com

Made in the USA
Coppell, TX
28 September 2021